Daniel Fast Dinner Recipes

Create Amazing Meals in No Time

Disclaimer

Contents

Salads, Sauces and Sidelines

Bread for Dinner
Servings: 10 people

Cooking Time: 45 minutes

Ingredients:

Allspice, ¼ tsp

Baking soda, 1 tsp

Cinnamon, 1 tsp

Coconut oil, 1 tsp

Extra virgin olive oil, ½ cup

Lemon juice, 1 tbsp

Pumpkin puree (preferably Libby's), 1 can

Raw agave nectar, ¾ cup

Salt, 1 tsp

Whole grain whole-wheat flour, 2 cups

Method:

1. Heat the oven at 350°F.
2. Grease the baking pan with coconut oil and sprinkle some flour on the top.
3. Mix agave nectar and olive oil in a bowl and add lemon juice and pumpkin juice to it too.
4. Now mix baking soda, flour, salt, and spices in another bowl.
5. Slowly add the ingredients of first bowl to the other one and mix properly.
6. Transfer the batter into the baking pan and keep it in the oven.
7. Bake it for 30 to 40 minutes and then take it out and enjoy!

Nutritional Value per Serving:

Calories 191.6

Carbohydrates 20.4 g

Cholesterol 0 g

Fats 12 g

Potato Salad
Servings: 8 people

Cooking Time: 45 minutes

Ingredients:

Onion (chopped), ½

Cider vinegar, 1 tbsp

Mixed herbs (chopped), ¼ cup

Potatoes (peeled and chopped), 3 lbs

Method:

1. Boil the potatoes, with some salt in the water. When they are completely boiled, drain the water and let them cool for a while.
2. After they cool off, peel their skin and mash them.
3. Add the remaining ingredients in the mashed potatoes mix them and then serve!

Nutritional Value per Serving:

Calories 200

Fats 6 g

Carbohydrates 33 g

Cholesterol less than 5 g

Crunchy Salad
Servings: 4 people

Cooking Time: 1 hour and 15 minutes

Ingredients:

Cider vinegar – 1/3 cup

Carrot (grated) – 1

Honey – Half tsp

Green bell pepper (chopper) – 1

Onion (chopped) – 1

Green cabbage (shredded) – 2 ½ lbs

Salt and pepper – As desired.

Method:

1. Combine all the chopped and shredded vegetables in a bowl.
2. Add salt, pepper, vinegar, and honey in the bowl too and mix well.
3. Cover the bowl and refrigerate it for an hour.
4. Serve cold and enjoy!

Nutritional Value per Serving:

Calories – 390

Fats – 24 g

Carbohydrates – 20 g

Cholesterol – 40 g

Garlic Loaded
Servings: 4 people

Cooking Time: 1 hour and 25 minutes

Ingredients:

Extra virgin olive oil – ½ cup

Thyme leaves – 1 tbsp

Coarse salt – A pinch

Garlic head – 1 lb

Method:

1. Set the oven at 400°F.
2. Separate the tops of the garlic heads, exposing the cloves.
3. Arrange all the sliced garlic heads in a greased baking dish.
4. Sprinkle salt and pepper on the cloves, and then pour some oil over them.
5. Wrap the baking dish with foil and bake it for at least half an hour.
6. You will see that the garlic clove shave softened.
7. After you have taken them out of the oven, squeeze their heads to push out the cloves.
8. Take them out in an air tight container and keep them aside.

Nutritional Value per Serving:

Calories – 410

Fats – 28 g

Carbohydrates – 39 g

Cholesterol – 0 g

Crispy Bites
Servings: 16 people

Cooking Time: 1 hour and 5 minutes

Ingredients:

Balsamic vinegar – 1 tsp

Extra virgin olive oil – 1 ½ cups

Fresh basil – Half bunch

Garlic cloves (minced) – 2

Plum tomatoes – 6

Italian bread – 1 loaf

Method:

1. Set the oven at 450°F.
2. On the other hand, boil tomatoes in a pot full of water and when they are done, drain the water, peel them off and remove their seeds.
3. After that roughly chop them into small pieces.
4. Mix basil leaves, salt, pepper and garlic in the tomatoes' bowl and stir them.
5. Cut the Italian bread into normal sized slices. Spread oil on one of their sides and then place them on a greased baking dish with the oil side pointing downwards.
6. After 5 minutes, take out the slices, flip them over and take spoonful of tomato mixture and transfer it on the oiled side of the bread.
7. Bake for another 6 to 10 minutes and then serve!

Nutritional Value per Serving:

Calories – 240

Fats – 21 g

Carbohydrates – 12 g

Cholesterol – 0 g

Meshed Avocado
Servings: 8 people

Cooking Time: 20 minutes

Ingredients:

Lime – 1

Coarse salt – As desired

Cilantro leaves (chopped) – ¼ cup

Jalapeno chilies (minced) – ½

Red onion (chopped) – ¼ cup

Avocado (ripe) - 3

Method:

1. Slice avocados in half, remove their soft part.
2. Mesh the avocado flesh with the help of spoon.
3. Add salt, cilantro, jalapeno and lime juice in the bowl too and combine.
4. Mix them with a light hand, making sure that it doesn't take goo-form.
5. Serve!

Nutritional Value per Serving:

Calories – 130

Fats – 11 g

Carbohydrates – 9 g

Cholesterol – 0 g

Easy to Make Tomato Sauce
Servings: 4 people

Cooking Time: 30 minutes

Ingredients:

Coarse salt – A pinch

Plum tomatoes – 3 lbs

Garlic (minced) – 1 tbsp

Extra virgin olive oil – 6 tbsp

Method:

1. Cook garlic in heated oil for 2 to 4 minutes.
2. When they start turning brown, add salt and tomatoes too.
3. Reduce the heat and let it cook at slow heat for 15 to 20 minutes.
4. Taste the sauce to see if you need any more salt or spices and then take it out in an air tight container.
5. You can refrigerate it for up to a week if you want.

Nutritional Value per Serving:

Calories – 240

Fats – 20 g

Carbohydrates – 14 g

Cholesterol – 0 g

Grill-y Scallops
Servings: 4 people

Cooking Time: 20 minutes

Ingredients:

Sea scallops – 20

Marinade – ½ cup

Marinade

Olive oil – ½ cup

Soy sauce – 2 tbsp

Yuzu (coarsely chopped) – 2 tbsp

Method:

1. Combine all the ingredients together and refrigerate them in an air tight container for around 2 weeks.
2. Take out 2 tablespoons of marinade and use the rest.
3. Place all the scallops in the marinade, rotating them around to cover the entire surface with the marinade.
4. Heat the grill at medium hot.
5. After that grill the scallops form all side until they are properly cooked.
6. When they are fully cooked, top them with the remaining marinade and serve!

Nutritional Value per Serving:

Calories – 110

Fats – 18 g

Carbohydrates – 16 g

Cholesterol – 0 g

Corn and Avocado Salad
Servings: 4 people

Cooking Time: 35 minutes

Ingredients:

Coarse salt – ½ tsp

Extra virgin olive oil – 1 tbsp

Fresh lime juice – 1tbsp

Fresh cilantro – ¼ cup

Avocado (sliced) – 1

Ear of corn – 4

Method:

1. Heat the grill at medium-high.
2. Grill al the corns for 15 minutes and after that separate them from the cob.
3. Take them out in a bowl and mix them with rest of the ingredients.
4. Stir them well and then serve!

Nutritional Value per Serving:

Calories – 110

Fats – 11 g

Carbohydrates – 5 g

Cholesterol – 0 g

Bakes Carrots
Servings: 4 people

Cooking Time: 40 minutes

Ingredients:

Salt and black pepper – A pinch

Olive oil

Agave nectar – 1 ½ tbsp

Balsamic vinegar – 1 ½ tbsp

Carrots – 1 lb

Method:

1. Heat the oven at 450°F.
2. Peel the carrots and then cut them into thin, vertical slices.
3. Mix balsamic vinegar and agave nectar in a bowl.
4. Arrange carrot slices in a greased baking dish and top them with the bowl ingredients.
5. Bake them for 20 minutes.
6. Then take them out, sprinkle salt and pepper and then serve!

Nutritional Value per Serving:

Calories – 620

Fats – 65 g

Carbohydrates – 11 g

Cholesterol – 0 g

Daniel Fast Soups and Stews

Mexican Bean Soup
Servings: 6

Cooking Time: 30 minutes

Ingredients

Black beans, 15 ounce (without sugar)

Frozen corn, 2 cups

Organic unsweetened salsa, 1 cup

Vegetable broth, 4 cups

Method

1) In a saucepan, combine all ingredients (altogether), and mix well.
2) Simmer for half an hour. Stir after every 4 to 5 minutes for extra smooth soupy texture.
3) Serve hot and enjoy the goodness of nature!

Nutritional Value per Serving

Carbohydrates 56 g

Facts: Calories 262

Protein 12.6 g

Total Fat 1.7 g

Soupy Pumpkins
Servings: 4

Cooking Time: 20 minutes

Ingredients

Cayenne pepper ½ teaspoon

Chopped chives (for garnishing)

Chopped onion, 1 (medium sized)

Curry powder, 1 tablespoon

Diced tomatoes, 14 ½ ounce (in form of juice)

Drained black beans, 15 ounce

Ground cumin, 1½ teaspoon

Olive oil, 2 tablespoons

Pumpkin puree, 15 ounce

Sea salt (to taste)

Soymilk, 1 cup

Vegetable stock, 3 cups

Method

1) In a saucepan, bring oil to heat.
2) Stir in onion and sauté it for about 5 minutes.
3) Now add tomatoes, black beans, vegetable broth, and pumpkin puree; and bring the mixture to a boil.
4) Once you see the boiling bubbles, reduce the heat and pour in soymilk, cayenne, salt, and curry powder. Keep stirring and simmer for 3 to 4 minutes.
5) Pour the soup into a serving bowl and garnish it with chives.
6) Enjoy hot!

Nutritional Value per serving

Calories 360

Carbohydrates 42g

Protein 18g

Total Fat 16g

Balsamic Vinegar Veggie Soup
Servings: 7

Cooking Time: 30 minutes

Ingredients

Balsamic vinegar, 1 Tbsp

Bay leaf, 1

Cannellini beans, 14 ounce (rinsed and drained)

Fresh spinach, 2 cups (stemmed and chopped)

Fresh thyme leaves, 2 tsp (chopped)

Frozen baby lima beans, 10 ounce

Large carrots, 3 (diced into half-inch thick slices)

Large parsnips, 2 (peeled and chopped into half inch pieces)

Minced garlic cloves, 6

Olive oil, 2 Tbsp

Onions, 2 small sized (diced into half-inch pieces)

Peel russet potatoes, 2 (cut into one-inch pieces)

Pepper (to taste)

Sea salt (to taste)

Sprig fresh rosemary, 1

Note: You may substitute cannellini beans with kidney beans.

Method

1) In large saucepan, bring oil to heat
2) Set the stove over medium-high flame.
3) Add in onions, parsnips, and carrots and sauté for about 5 to 6 minutes. Make sure the vegetables are soft before you proceed further.
4) Stir in minced garlic and cook for 30 seconds.
5) Now pour in vegetable broth, potatoes, bay leaf, thyme, and rosemary.
6) Reduce the heat to low, after the first boil.
7) Cover the pan and cook for another 10 minutes.

8) With the help of a spoon or spatula, take out the rosemary and bay leaf.
9) Take out 1 cup of soup of soup and 3 cups of vegetable from the saucepan and pour it all in a food processor.
10) Whirl until a smooth puree is formed.
11) Pour back the puree into the saucepan along with lima beans, spinach, and cannellini beans.
12) Increase the heat and simmer for 5 to 7 minutes.
13) Finally add in a pinch of pepper, salt, and balsamic.
14) Serve hot!

Nutritional Value per Serving

Calories 217

Carbohydrates 38.6 g

Protein 6.9 g

Total Fat 4.4 g

Peas and Carrot Stew
Serving: 8

Cooking Time: 4 hours

Ingredients

Ground cumin ¼ teaspoons

Rinsed split peas, 2 cups

Diced onion, 1 (medium sized)

Minced garlic cloves, 2

Hot water, 6 cups

Black pepper, ¼ teaspoon

Diced carrots, 1 cup

Dried basil, ½ teaspoon

Sliced celery, 1 cup

Cayenne pepper, (a pinch of it)

Dried marjoram, ½ teaspoon

Sea salt 1 teaspoon

Method

1) In a slow cooker, combine all of the above ingredients.
2) For about 3 minutes, mix well over low heat.
3) Cover the cover and let the soup cook for about 3 hours. Before serving, check if the peas are tender and cooked thoroughly.
4) Serve and enjoy the hot stew!

Nutritional Value per Serving

Calories 81.4

Carbohydrates 15.5g

Protein 5g

Total Fat 0.3g

Mix Vegetable Soup
Servings: 8

Cooking Time: 6 hours

Ingredients

Brown rice, 1 cup (cooked)

Carrots, 3 (diced into thick slices)

Celery, 4 stalks (chopped)

Diced tomatoes, 15 ounce (in form of juice)

Diced yellow onion, 1 (medium sized)

Green beans, 2 cups (cut into small pieces)

Green cabbage, 1 head (cored and cut into slices)

Italian herbs, 2 tablespoons

Minced garlic cloves, 5

Olive oil, ½ cup

Pepper (to taste)

Red bell pepper, 1 (chopped)

Sea Salt (to taste)

Vegetable stock, 8 cups

Method

1) In a slow cooker, combine all the above listed ingredients and mix well.
2) Cover the cooker, and cook the entire mixture for about 5 hours. Depending on the cooking heat, it may require up to 6 hours also.
3) Serve hot and enjoy the vegetable delight.

Nutritional Value per Serving

Calories 251

Carbohydrates 27 g

Protein 4.2 g

Total Fat 15 g

Butternut Squash Curry Soup
Servings: 4

Cooking Time: 40 minutes

Ingredients

Butternut squash, 1 large piece

Chopped green onions, ¼ cup

Curry powder, 2 tablespoons

Olive oil, 3 tablespoons

Pepper (to taste)

Salt (to taste)

Vegetable bouillon cube, 1

Water, 2 cups

Method

1) Dissolve the vegetable bouillon cube in water and set aside.
2) Cut the deseeded and peeled squash into one inch cubes
3) Boil the squash cubes in a saucepan filled with water. Once it is boiled, leave only 2 tablespoons of water in the pan while discarding the remaining.
4) Using a potato masher, mash the boil squash.
5) Add in green onions, oil, and curry powder and mix vigorously.
6) Also, stir in salt and pepper as per your personal taste and preferences.
7) Start pouring in the bouillon broth. Do not add it all together. Add in small quantities and stop where you feel the soup will lose its consistency.
8) Simmer for another 10 to 15 minutes.
9) Enjoy this delicious soup!

Nutritional Value per Serving

Calories 211

Carbohydrates 26g

Protein 3.3g

Total Fat 12g

Tomato Juice Corn Soup
Servings: 8

Cooking Time: 15 minutes

Ingredients

Canned black beans, 15½ ounce (drained)

Canned corn, 15 ½ oz. (drained)

Diced tomatoes & chilies, 14 ½ ounce

Medium sized onion, 1 chopped

Pepper (to taste)

Sea salt (to taste)

Tomato juice, 4 cups

Vegetable stock, 2 cups

Preparation Method

1) Combine all the ingredients in a cooking pot.
2) Cover it and cook the soup for 15 to 20 minutes. Make sure all ingredients are heated and cooked through.
3) Serve hot and enjoy this yummylicious soup.

Nutritional Value per Serving

Calories 224

Carbohydrates 44.4 g

Protein 12.3 g

Total Fat 1.2 g

Jalapeno Soup with Beans and Tomatoes
Servings: 6

Cooking Time: 30 minutes

Ingredients

Black beans, 30 ounce (rinsed and drained)

Chopped onion, 2 medium

Diced tomatoes with liquid, 15 ounce

Finely chopped celery, ¾ cup

Ground black pepper (to taste)

Ground cumin, 1 teaspoon

Jalapeño pepper, 2 teaspoon (finely chopped)

Minced garlic, 1 teaspoon

Olive oil, 1 tablespoon

Red pepper flakes (to taste)

Salt (to taste)

Water, 2 cups

Method

1) Bring oil to heat in a non-stick skillet
2) Set the stove over medium heat
3) When the oil is hot, stir in garlic and onion, and cook for about 2 minutes.
4) Add in jalapeno pepper and celery and cook for another 2 minutes.
5) Turn off the heat and set aside.
6) Separately, in a food processor, combine water with, half of the diced tomatoes and half of the black beans.
7) Pulse once or twice to make a smooth puree of ingredients
8) Turn on the stove over medium heat
9) Transfer the entire puree to a large saucepan along with the sautéed onion mixture, remaining tomatoes, and remaining beans. Mix well.
10) Add in a bit of salt, pepper, pepper flakes, and cumin; and cover the pan for 5 minutes.
11) Now reduce the heat and cook another 15 to 20 minutes, or until the desired texture of soup is ready.

12) Serve hot and enjoy the Jalapeno Soup!

Nutritional Value per Serving

Calories 163.5

Carbohydrates 26 g

Protein 8.8 g

Total Fat 3 g

Mushroom Soup
Servings: 6

Cooking Time: 40 minutes

Ingredients

Diced onions, 2 medium sized

Dill 1½ teaspoon

Flour, 3 tablespoon

Ground black pepper (a pinch of it for taste)

Lemon juice, 2 teaspoon

Mushrooms, 1 lb (cut into slices)

Oil, 3 tablespoons (divided)

Paprika, 1 tablespoon

Soy sauce, 2 tablespoon

Soymilk, 1 cup

Vegetable stock, 2 cups

Method

1) In a soup pot, bring 1 tablespoon of oil to heat over medium-high flame.
2) Sauté onions until it is tender
3) Add in paprika, dill, and mushrooms to the pot. Cook for another 5 minutes and the pour in vegetable stock and soy sauce. Reduce the heat and simmer for 15 minutes. Make sure you cover the pot for additional aroma and taste.
4) Separately, in another saucepan, heat the remaining 2 tablespoons of oil. Once the oil is hot, add in flour, and keep stirring for 1 minute. Dispense in soymilk and whisk so that there are no lumps.
5) Cook until it is slightly thickened.
6) Now combine paprika-mushroom mixture into the smooth saucy soymilk and simmer for 15 to 20 minutes.
7) Add lemon juice and serve hot!

Nutritional Value per Serving

Calories 111.7

Carbohydrates 11g,

Protein 3.9g

Total Fat 7g,

Carrot Soup
Servings: 6

Cooking Time: 1 hour

Ingredients

Bean soup mix, ½ lb

Chopped onions, ½ cup

Diced carrots, ½ cup

Ground black pepper (to taste)

Kosher salt (to taste)

Water, 3 ½ cups

Method

1) In a cooking pot, combine water along with bean mix, onions, and carrots.
2) Over low heat, bring it to boil.
3) After the first boil, reduce the heat, cover the pot, and let it cook for 1 hour.
4) Season the soup with salt and pepper as per your own taste.
5) Serve hot and enjoy this low calorie soup!

Nutritional Value per Serving

Calories 129.4

Carbohydrates 22g

Protein 8.3g

Total Fat 5g

Main Course

Italian Brown Rise with Mixed Vegetables
Servings: 8

Cooking Time: 1 hour

Ingredients

Brown rice, 4 cups (cooked)

Diced tomatoes, 30 ounce

Extra virgin olive oil, 2 tablespoons

Green bell peppers, 8

Italian seasoning, 3 tablespoons

Mixed vegetable, 6 cups

Tomato Sauce, 30 ounce (divided)

White onion, 1 (medium sized)

Method

1) Preheat the oven at 350F°
2) Cut the tops of the washed and deseeded green peppers.
3) Separately, sauté mixed vegetables and onions over medium-high heat.
4) Once all vegetables are tender, add in one half of tomato sauce and brown rice.
5) Keep stirring for one minute.
6) Now stuff the veggie mixture in the peppers.
7) Carefully line the peppers on a casserole dish.
8) Place the dish in the oven and bake it for 45 minutes. Make sure pepper crispy yet a bit tender. If it becomes too crisp, it will lose its natural juiciness.
9) Meanwhile, in a wok, combine diced tomatoes, Italian seasoning, and the remaining tomato sauce and cook until tomatoes are heated through.
10) Take out the peppers and pour equal amounts of tomato sauce on each piece.

Serve hot and enjoy the dinner!

Nutritional Value per Serving

Calories 537

Carbohydrates 103.5 g

Protein 13.5 g

Total Fat 8.5 g

Mexican Beans Delight
Servings: 8

Cooking Time: 20 minutes

Ingredients

Black beans or pinto beans, 14 ounce or 1 can (rinsed and drained)

Chili powder, 1 tablespoon

Chopped fresh cilantro, ¼ cup

Chopped leek, 1

Extra virgin olive oil, 2 tablespoon

Ground cumin, 1 teaspoon

Medium sized carrot, 1 (diced)

Minced garlic, 1 tablespoon

Red bell pepper, 1 (chopped and seeded)

Vegetable broth, 4 cups

Zucchinis, 2 (cut in small cubes)

Method

1) In a large skillet, bring oil to heat
2) Set stove at medium-high flame and sauté chili powder, leek, cumin, and garlic for about 4 minutes.
3) Stir in zucchini, carrots, and bell pepper and cook for another 5 minutes.
4) Now pour in broth to the skillet and bring the mixture to a boil.
5) Once you see the boiling bubbles, reduce the heat, and add beans to it.
6) Cook for 10 to 15 more minutes and then stir in cilantro.

Enjoy this mouthwatering dinner meal with family and friends!

Nutritional Value per Serving

Calories 255.8

Carbohydrates 43 g

Protein 13 g

Total Fat 4.3 g

Italian Cabbage Rolls with Tomato Sauce
Servings: 6

Cooking Time: 40 minutes

Ingredients

Cabbage leaves, 12 large

Chopped fresh parsley, 2 tablespoons

Cooked brown rice, 1 cup

Crushed oregano, 1 teaspoon

Diced onion, 1 cup

Grated carrot, 1 cup

Italian herbs, 1 teaspoon

Mushrooms, ½ lb (sliced)

Olive oil, 2 tablespoons

Pepper, ¼ teaspoon

Salt, ½ teaspoon

Tomato sauce, 15 ounce

Vegetable oil (for greasing the pan)

White beans, 15 ounce (washed and drained)

Method

1) Preheat the oven at 350F°
2) Using a few drops of vegetable oil, grease a 2-quart baking pan.
3) In a large sauce pan, bring water to boil. Soak the cabbages in the boiling water and cook for 2 to 3 minutes. Once the cabbage is softened, drain the water and water for it to cool down.
4) Meanwhile, in another non-stick pan, bring oil to heat, and sauté mushrooms and onions until tender.
5) Add in carrots, parsley, oregano, salt, pepper beans, and brown rice and mix well.

6) Take equal portion of rice and vegetable mixture and place it in each cabbage leave.
7) Carefully roll up the leaves in a way that the stuffing does not come out during baking.
8) Line all cabbage rolls in the greased baking pan and cover it with foil paper.
9) Place the dish into the oven and bake for half an hour.
10) Meanwhile, in another saucepan, reheat the tomato sauce and Italian herbs.
11) Enjoy hot cabbage rolls with delicious Italian tomato sauce!

Nutritional Value per Serving

Calories 184

Carbohydrates 29 g

Protein 7 g

Total Fat 5.5 g

Pearl Barley Casserole
Servings: 4

Cooking Time: 1 hour

Ingredients

Black beans, 15 ounce (rinsed and drained)

Chopped green pepper, ½ cup

Chopped onion, 1 cup

Fresh mushroom, 2 cups (cut into slices)

Ground black pepper (to taste)

Olive oil cooking spray

Salt (to taste)

Sunflower seeds, 3 tablespoons

Uncooked pearl barley, 1 cup

Vegetable broth, 1¼-cup

Water, 1¼ cup

Method

1) Preheat the oven at 350F°
2) Spread the uncooked pearl barley on a baking sheet and bake it for about 8 minutes.
3) Take out the lightly browned barley in a saucepan. Do not switch off the oven.
4) Pour water and broth into the saucepan and bring it to a boil.
5) Once you see the boiling bubbles on the surface, reduce the heat, and cover the saucepan. Cook for another 20 minutes or until liquid is absorbed by barley.
6) Meanwhile, spray oil onto a non-stick pan and heat it over medium coat the insides of a nonstick skillet with cooking spray and heat eat it.
7) Add in onions, green pepper, and mushrooms and sauté until all vegetables are tender. It might take about 5 to 10 minutes.
8) Now stir in beans and cooked barley.
9) Season it with salt and pepper (as per your own taste and lifestyle preferences)
10) Using cooking spray, grease a casserole-baking dish
11) Shift the mixture into the greased baking dish, cover the dish with foil paper, and bake it for half an hour.

12) Uncover the dish, sprinkle sunflower seeds on top, and again bake it for 5 minutes.

13) Serve hot!

Nutritional Value per Serving

Calories 445.6

Carbohydrates 71 g

Protein 18.4 g

Total Fat 12 g

Sautéed Tofu and Spinach
Servings: 4

Cooking Time: 15 minutes

Ingredients

Chopped onion, 1 medium sized

Chopped tomatoes, 2

Curry powder, 1 teaspoon

Extra virgin olive oil, 1 teaspoon

Firm tofu, 1 block or 340 grams (pressed, drained, and crumbled)

Fresh spinach, 1 bunch

Ground black pepper (to taste)

Ground cumin, ½ teaspoon

Ground turmeric, ½ teaspoon

Minced garlic cloves, 3

Salt (to taste)

Method

1) In a non-stick pan, bring oil to heat.
2) Sauté garlic and onion for about 5 minutes
3) Once the onion is tender, stir in salt, pepper, turmeric, cumin, curry powder, tofu, and tomatoes. Over medium heat, cook for 5 to 7 minutes, or until tofu is thoroughly cooked.
4) Finally, add in spinach and cook no more than 5 minutes.
5) Enjoy it hot!

Nutritional Value per Serving

Calories 173.6

Carbohydrates 13 g

Protein 15.5 g

Total Fat 9 g

Picante Burger Patties
Servings: 8

Cooking Time: 15 minutes

Ingredients

Brown rice cakes, 1 cup or about 2 cakes (crushed)

Canned red kidney beans, 16 ounce (drained & mashed)

Carrot, 1 medium sized (steamed & mashed)

Chopped onion, 1 cup

Ground black pepper, ½ teaspoon

Picante sauce, 2 tablespoons (preferably organic or homemade)

Pinch of chili powder

Salt, ½ teaspoon

Whole-wheat flour, ½ cup

Method

1) Preheat the oven at 450F°
2) In a large bowl, combine all the ingredients and mix well. If it is too stiff, you can add a little bit more of picante sauce. Similarly, to make it more firm, pour in some more flour. Remember that picante sauce is quite spicy; do not pour in too much of it unless you are habitual of eating spicy food.
3) Divide the mixture into 8 equal portions and carefully 8 patties.
4) Place them on a baking sheet, and bake for about 12 to 15 minutes.
5) Treat your taste buds with these delicious burger patties. Serve with burger buns or whole wheat bread for maximum taste.

Nutritional Value per Serving

Calories 103

Carbohydrates 19.7 g

Protein 4.8 g

Total Fat 0.5 g

Lentils with BBQ Spices
Servings: 4

Cooking Time: 30 minutes

Ingredients

Chopped fresh cilantro, 1 bunch

Chopped green chili, 1 (seeded)

Cinnamon stick, 1 (3 inches)

Creamed coconut, 100 grams

Crushed garlic cloves, 4

Diced onion, 1 large

Hot water, 4 ¼ cups

Lemon, 1

Mango relish, 1 tablespoon

Olive oil, 1 tablespoon

Red lentils, 450 grams (rinsed and drained)

Salt (to taste)

Tikka masala curry paste, 2 tablespoons

Tomato paste, 2 tablespoon

Method

1) In a large non-stick pan, bring olive oil to heat and sauté garlic and onion, until tender.
2) Separately, in a large bowl, dissolve creamed coconut in hot water and pour it in the pan in which you just sautéed garlic and onion.
3) Stir in mango relish, tomato paste, cinnamon stick, lentils, curry powder, and half lemon. Mix well. Simmer the mixture for about 15 minutes. It should become think and creamy.
4) Using a spoon or spatula, discard the cinnamon stick and lemon.
5) Season it with cilantro, salt, and remaining lime juice.
6) Serve hot!

Nutritional Value per serving

Calories 321

Carbohydrates 26.4 g

Protein 8 g

Total Fat 22.3 g

Veggie-Broccoli Crumble

Servings: 8

Cooking Time: 40 minutes

Ingredients

Broccoli florets, 4 cups

Cauliflower floret, 2 cups

Chopped onion, 1 ½ cup

Curry powder, 5 teaspoon

Fresh cilantro, ½ cup

Ground cumin, 2 teaspoon

Large potatoes, 5 (peeled and diced into 1-inch cubes)

Low fat evaporated milk, 2 cups

Plum tomatoes, 2 cups (diced and seeded)

Red pepper flakes, ¼ teaspoon

Thinly sliced carrots, 4 cups

Vegetable oil cooking spray

Method

1) Spray the vegetable oil on a non-stick skillet and heat it over medium-high flame.
2) Sauté onion for 7 to 10 minutes or until it is softened.
3) Once the onion is tender, stir in red pepper flakes and curry powder, and cook for about a minute on low heat.
4) Pour in milk and bring the mixture to a boil.
5) Stir in tomatoes and potatoes into the boiling blend.
6) Now cover the pan and simmer for approximately 12 to 15 minutes. Stir occasionally to makes sure everything mixes well.
7) Add in broccoli, carrots, and cauliflower, and continue cooking for about 8 minutes.
8) Use salt and pepper for seasoning
9) Garnish it with fresh cilantro and enjoy the meal!

Nutritional Value per Serving

Calories 212

Carbohydrates 33 g

Protein 5.2 g

Total Fat 3.6 g

Moroccan Style Chickpeas
Servings: 5

Cooking Time: 15 minutes

Ingredients

¾-cup vegetable broth, Half cup

Canned chickpeas, 15 ½ ounce (drained and rinsed)

Chopped onions, ½ cup

Extra virgin olive oil, 1 tablespoon

Green chilies with tomatoes, 14 ½ ounce or 1 can

Ground black pepper (to taste)

Ground coriander, 1 tablespoon

Ground cumin, 1 tablespoon

Ground ginger, ½ tablespoon

Minced garlic cloves, 2

Salt (to taste)

Method

1) In a non-stick skillet, bring oil to heat over medium flame
2) In hot oil, sauté garlic and onion for approximately 3 minutes
3) Add in cumin, ginger, and ground coriander and continue cooking until onion is tender.
4) Then pour in vegetable broth along with green-chilled-tomatoes and chickpeas. Cover the skillet and cook for another 10 to 15 minutes.
5) Serve hot and eat fresh!

Nutritional Value per Serving

Calories 173

Carbohydrates 29 g

Protein 6 g

Total Fat 4.4 g

Golden Cornbread Pie
Servings: 8

Cooking Time: 1 hour and 15 minutes

Ingredients

Baking powder, ½ teaspoon

Basil, 1 tablespoon

Canned green chilies, 4 ounce (chopped)

Canned tomato, 14 ½ ounce (diced)

Chili powder, 3 tablespoon

Chopped onion, 1 medium sized

Cooked pinto beans, 4 cups (mashed)

Corn kernels, 2 cups

Cornmeal, 1 ½ cups

Garlic powder, 1 teaspoon

Green bell pepper, 1(diced)

Ground black pepper (to taste)

Oregano, 1 teaspoon

Salt (to taste)

Salt, ¼ teaspoon

Tomato sauce, 1 cup

Vegetable oil cooking spray

Vegetable oil, 2 tablespoons

Water, 3 cups

Whole-wheat flour, ½ cup

Method

1) In a large pot, bring oil to heat.
2) Over medium flame, sauté onions for approximately 8 to 10 minutes
3) Stir in tomato sauce, green pepper, basil, chili powder, corns, oregano, green chilies, tomatoes, salt, and pepper; and cook for about 5 minutes.
4) Stir the mashed beans and mix well. Cook for 10 more minutes and keep stirring occasionally.
5) Remove the pan from the stove and set aside.
6) Preheat the oven at 350F°
7) Meanwhile, in another saucepan, combine whole-wheat flour with salt, cornmeal, and baking powder. Mix all ingredients well.
8) Cover the pan and cook until mixture thickens.
9) Take out a 9X3 baking dish and coat it oil using a cooking spray.
10) Start making the layers by first pouring in half of the cornmeal mixture. Make next layer with bean mixture and then finally lay the third layers using the remaining cornmeal mixture.
11) Place it in the preheated oven, and bake for approximately 40 to 45 minutes.
12) Serve the golden cornbread pie!

Nutritional Value per serving

Calories 305

Carbohydrates 56.8 g

Protein 11 g

Total Fat 5.4 g

Beans with Green Bell Peppers
Servings: 12

Cooking Time: 4 hours

Ingredients

Canned diced tomatoes, 14 ½ ounce

Canned kidney beans, 15 ounce (undrained)

Canned tomato paste, 14 ½ ounce

Chili powder (to taste)

Chopped green bell peppers, 1

Chopped green chili, 4 ounce (canned)

Chopped onions, 5 small

Diced celery with leaves, 4 stalks

Extra virgin olive oil, 3 tablespoons

Ground cinnamon, ¼ teaspoon

Ground cumin, ¼ teaspoon

Minced garlic, 4 teaspoon

Salt & pepper (to taste)

Undrained black beans, 15 ounce (canned)

Yellow soy beans 5 cups (cooked) – Do not throw away the cooking liquid

Method

1) In a nonstick pan, bring oil to heat.
2) Over medium flame, sauté green peppers, celery, onions, and garlic for about 7 to 10 minutes or until onion are tender.
3) Transfer the mixture to a slow cooker along with all other ingredients.
4) To make the curry or paste think or thin, add appropriate amount of liquid from soybeans.
5) Cover the cooker and cook for about 3 to 4 hours.
6) Serve hot and enjoy a healthy Daniel fast dinner!

Nutritional Value per Serving

Calories 313

Carbohydrates 40.6 g

Protein 18.7 g

Total Fat 9.5 g

A Veggie Delight for the Love of Thai Food
Servings: 8

Cooking Time: 15 minutes

Ingredients

Chopped broccoli, 2 cups

Fresh green beans, 1 ½ cups (cut into slices)

Green bell peppers, 2 (diced into slices)

Lemongrass, 4 stems (cut into thin slices)

Limejuice, 4 tablespoons

Minced garlic cloves, 8

Minced green chilies, 4

Red bell peppers, 2 (diced into slices)

Salt (to taste)

Sesame oil, 6 tablespoon

Thinly sliced carrots, 1 ½ cups

Tofu, 1 block (cut into small cubes)

Method

1) In a large wok, bring oil to heat
2) Sauté tofu cubes for approximately 5 minutes or until lightly golden browned.
3) Add in all vegetables and cook for five more minutes.
4) Now add all the remaining ingredients and continue cooking for 3 to 4 minutes. Keep stirring to make sure all ingredients are mixed well.
5) Enjoy the delightful Thai dinner with brown or plain rice.

Nutritional Value per Serving

Calories 461

Carbohydrates 22 g

Total Fat 28 g

Protein 30 g

Lentil and Mushroom Patty Cakes
Servings: 6

Cooking Time: 30 minutes

Ingredients

Cajun seasoning, 1 teaspoon

Chopped garlic cloves, 2

Chopped mushrooms, 6

Chopped onion, 1 medium sized

Cooked lentils, 2 cups

Grated carrot, 1 medium sized

Ground black pepper (to taste)

Italian mixed herbs, ½ teaspoon

Olive oil for frying (you may substitute it with any other vegetable oil)

Salt (to taste)

Soft tofu, 1 cup (cut into 1-inch cubes)

Method

1) In large wok, bring oil to heat
2) Sauté the mushroom in vegetable or olive oil for about 4 to 5 minutes
3) Then add onion, garlic, and carrots and continue cooking for five more minutes.
4) Now pour in tofu along with herbs, lentils, and Cajun seasoning. Fry for 8 to 10 minutes. Make sure you keep stirring so that all spices and herbs are mixed thoroughly.
5) Season it salt and pepper as per your own taste.
6) Carefully divide the mixture into 6 equal parts.
7) Use your hands to form patties or small cakes. Do not worry if the patties are not as round as the ones you find in the market, this one certainly tastes better. As you continue practicing, you will surely get hold of it.
8) Fry the patties in oil for approximately 4 minutes each side. Depending on the heat of the stove, it may require a minute more or less.
9) Serve hot and enjoy the dinner!

Nutritional Value per Serving

Calories 136

Carbohydrates 17 g

Protein 9.5 g

Total Fat 4 g

Potato and Spinach Curry
Servings: 4

Cooking Time: 30 minutes

Ingredients

Baby spinach leaves, 180 grams

Cauliflower, 1(diced into florets)

Chopped onion, 1 medium sized

Chopped tomatoes, 14 ounce (canned)

Crushed garlic cloves, 3

Curry paste, 3 tablespoons

Diced red chilies, 2 (seeded)

Peeled potatoes, 300 grams (cut into small chunks or thin wedges)

Vegetable broth, 1 ¾ cups

Vegetable oil cooking spray

Method

1) Use a cooking spray to coat a large skillet and bring oil to heat over medium flame.
2) Sauté garlic and onions until tender
3) Add in red chilies and cook for another two minutes, while stirring consistently.
4) Then add in curry paste, cauliflower florets, and potato chunks and mix well.
5) Cook for 4 to 5 minutes and then stir in broth and tomatoes.
6) Once the mixture comes to a boil, cover the skillet and simmer for about 18 to 20 minutes.
7) Finally add in spinach and serve hot!

Nutritional Value per Serving

Calories 188

Carbohydrates 32.7 g

Protein 8.4 g

Total Fat 3.7 g

Curried Chickpeas
Servings: 4

Cooking Time: 15 minutes

Ingredients

Chopped onions, 1 cup

Cayenne pepper, 1 tablespoon

Salt, 1 teaspoon

Cumin seeds, 1 teaspoon

Canned chickpeas, 2 cups

Olive oil or canola oil, 2 tablespoons

Method

1) In a non-stick pan, bring oil to heat and sauté onions until caramelized or browned.
2) Add in chickpeas, salt and pepper and cook until thoroughly cooked.
3) Enjoy this simple yet delicious dinner meal with plain or brown rice.

Nutritional Value per Serving

Calories 159.4

Carbohydrates 22 g

Protein 6.6 g

Total Fat 4.7 g

Serrano Dinner Burritos
Servings: 4

Cooking Time: 10 minutes

Ingredients

Chopped fresh cilantro, ½ cup

Chopped onion, ½ cup

Cooked brown rice, 2 cups

Extra firm tofu, 2 cups (crumbled)

Extra virgin olive oil, 2 tablespoons

Fresh lime juice, 2 teaspoon

Minced garlic cloves, 1

Roma tomatoes, 3 (seeded and chopped)

Salt, 2 teaspoons

Serrano chilies, 4 (seeded and finely chopped)

Whole-wheat tortillas, 4

Method

1) Heat olive oil in a large non-stick skillet.
2) Sauté garlic and onions until ingredients are tender.
3) Add in tofu and brown rice and keep stirring for 4 minutes or until they are thoroughly mixed.
4) Then stir in Serrano chilies, tomatoes, and cilantro and continue cooking for 5 minutes.
5) Sprinkle over lime juice just before serving.
6) Scoop out equal portions of mixture on tortillas and enjoy your dinner with family and friends!

Nutritional Value per Serving

Calories 381.3

Carbohydrates 54 g

Total Fat 14 g

Protein 13.5 g

Chickpeas with Coconut Curry
Servings: 4

Cooking Time: 1 hour

Ingredients

Chopped cilantro leaves, 4 tablespoons

Chopped tomatoes, 200g (canned)

Coconut cream, 200ml

Curry paste, 2 tablespoons

Drained chickpeas, 14 ½ ounce or 1 can

Finely diced onion, 1 large

Ground almonds, 2 tablespoons

Handful of spinach

Mango chutney, 1 tablespoon

Minced garlic cloves, 4

Olive oil, 1 tablespoon

Peeled potatoes, 3 large (cut into 1-inch chunks)

Peeled sweet potato, 1 large (cut into one-inch chunks)

Salt (to taste)

Squeezed lemon, 1

Tomato paste, 1 tablespoon

Vegetable stock, 2 cups

Method

1) In a non-stick skillet, bring oil to heat over medium flame.
2) Add a pinch of salt along with onions and garlic to the hot oil and sauté for about 5 minutes.
3) Once the onions are translucent, add the onions and curry paste and keep stirring for another 2 to 3 minutes.

4) Now add chickpeas, potatoes, and all the remaining ingredients, except for the spinach.
5) As soon as the mixture comes to a boil, reduce the heat, cover the pan, and simmer for about 45 minutes. Occasionally stir to make sure ingredients blend well with the spices.
6) Just when you are ready to serve, sprinkle over a handful of spinach and stir for a minute or two.
7) Enjoy this delicious dinner meal with whole wheat tortillas or brown rice.

Nutritional Value per Serving

Calories 456

Carbohydrates 76.6 g

Total Fat 14 g

Protein 10.4 g

Desserts

Baked Pears
Servings: 4

Cooking Time: 30 minutes

Ingredients

Ground cinnamon (a pinch of it)

Unpeeled and thinly sliced pears (about 2 cups slices)

Unsweetened pear juice, 1 cup

Method

1) Preheat the oven at 300F°
2) On a square baking sheet, line the pear slices
3) In a separate bowl, combine cinnamon and pear juice, and pour it over the lined pears in the baking dish.
4) Place it in the oven for about 15 minutes.
5) Bring the dish out of the oven, stir the mixture, and again place it in the oven for 15 minutes.

To delight your taste buds, serve warm!

Nutritional Value per Serving

Calories 80

Carbohydrates 21.3 g

Protein 1.1 g

Total Fat 0.3 g

Crushed Fruity Ice
Servings: 5 to 6

Cooking Time: 5 minutes

Ingredients

Orange juice, ½ cup

Peaches, 1 cup (canned or frozen)

Strawberries, 1 cup (frozen)

Cantaloupe cubes, 2 cups

Sugar, 2 teaspoon

Pineapple chunks, 2/3 cup

Ice cubes (Minimum 5, Maximum 8) choose as per taste

Method

1) Pulse all ingredients in a food processor.
2) Once all the ingredients are thoroughly blended, pour the mixture into serving bowls.
3) Since it is a cold dessert, it is best to make it only at the time of serving
4) Enjoy the fruity icy dessert.

Nutritional Value per Serving

Calories 1.9

Carbohydrates 27 g

Protein 1.5 g

Total Fat 0.1 g

Brown Rice and Pineapple Pudding
Servings: 2

Cooking Time: 30 minutes

Ingredients

Fresh Pineapple (2 diced slices)

Ground cinnamon, ¼ teaspoon

Long Grain brown rice (1 ½ cups cooked)

Low fat soy milk, 1 cup (vanilla flavored)

Raisins, 2 ounce

Method

1) In a saucepan, combine all ingredients.
2) On medium heat, simmer for about 30 minutes.
3) Let it cool for a while and enjoy the delicious dessert with family and friends!

Nutritional Value per Serving

Calories 199.7

Carbohydrates 45.6 g

Protein 4.2 g

Total Fat 2.4 g

Pecan and Apple Surprise
Servings: 4 to 5

Cooking Time: 60 minutes

Ingredients

Chopped pecans, ½ cup

Half cup Oat Groats

Medium sized apples, 3 (sliced with skin-on)

Nutmeg and ground cinnamon (to taste)

Orange juice, ½ cup

Raisins, 3 ounce

Water, 1 cup

Method

1) Preheat the oven at 300F°
2) In a bowl, pour on orange juice, water, and oats.
3) Now stir in pecans, nutmeg, sliced apples, and raisins.
4) Grease a baking pan
5) Transfer the mixture the greased pan.
6) Cook in the oven for 60 minutes or until oats are cooked
7) Enjoy the apple treat with a loved one!

Nutritional Value per Serving

Calories 252.4

Carbohydrates 41.6 g

Protein 4.4 g

Total Fat 10 g

Peanut Butter Cookies
Yields: 10 to 12 cookies

Cooking Time: 15 minutes

Ingredients

Whole-wheat flour, ½ cup

Ripe banana, half

Ground cinnamon, ½ teaspoon

Dry Quaker oats, ½ cup

Ground ginger, 1/8 teaspoon

Natural peanut butter, 2 tablespoon

Raisins, ½ cup (divided)

Natural applesauce, 4 ounce (unsweetened)

Water, ¼ cup

Method

1) Preheat the oven at 300F°
2) In a food processor, combine banana, raisins, and water; and pulse until a well-blended mixture is formed
3) Pour the mixture into a bowl and add in the remaining ingredients
4) Roll it in your hands to form 10 to 12 small balls (the number of cookies depend on the size)
5) Shape each ball into a cookie and place each of them in a greased baking sheet. Make sure all pieces are at least an inch apart from one another.
6) Place the baking dish into the preheated oven and bake the cookies for about 10 to 12 minutes.
7) Call your friends over for a tea party and enjoy the delicious cookies.

Nutritional Value per Serving

Calories 88

Carbohydrates 13 g

Protein 2.6 g

Total Fat 3 g

Frozen Banana Delight
Servings: 4

Cooking Time: 5 minutes

Ingredients

Cocoa powder (for garnishing)

Maple syrup (for garnishing)

Peeled frozen bananas, 4 (sliced)

Method

1) In a food processor, put the frozen bananas and pulse until a smooth mixture is formed
2) Transfer the blended fruit to a bowl and place it in the freezer for 20 minutes.
3) Make servings by scooping it into bowls.
4) Sprinkle cocoa powder and pour some maple syrup onto each serving
5) Serve immediately and enjoy the fruity fresh flavor of banana with family!

Nutritional Value per Serving

Calories 105.4

Carbohydrates 27 g

Protein 1.3 g

Total Fat 0.4 g

Apple and Oat Cookies

Yields: 10 to 12cookies

Cooking Time: 4 hours

Ingredients

Apple, 1 (chopped)

Crushed almonds, ¾ cup

Dates, 5 (pitted)

Dried cranberries, 1/3 cup

Oats flour, 1 cups

Orange juice, ½ cup

Roasted cashew nuts, ¼ cups (grounded)

Method

1) In a large bowl, combine all ingredients, except for cashew nuts.
2) Mix well, and then use the mixture to form cookies. Do not worry if your cookies aren't round or even.
3) Coast each piece with grounded cashew nuts. Feel free sprinkle a little bit of oats flour to settle the final shape of the cookies.
4) Carefully place the cookies in dehydrator for 3 to 4 hours. You may leave it for extra half an hour to attain the desired texture.
5) Enjoy the chunky cookies with a loved one!

Nutritional Value per Serving

Calories 151

Carbohydrates 28.7 g

Protein 3.4 g

Total Fat 5.8 g

Avocado Gelato with Coconuts
Servings: 12

Cooking Time: 5 minutes

Ingredients

Almond milk, ½ cup (unsweetened)

Avocados, 3

Chocolate-flavored liquid, 1 dropper

Cocoa powder, 2 tablespoons

Coconut butter, ¼ cup

Coconut flakes, 3 tablespoons (unsweetened)

Honey or rice syrup for vegans, ¼ cup

Sugar-free chocolate protein powder, 3 tablespoons

Method

1) In a food processor, blend all ingredients except for coconut flakes. Pulse until the mixture becomes creamy and smooth. Remember, the paste should be very think.
2) Scoop a tablespoon of mixture and place it flat onto a cookie sheet.
3) Sprinkle coconut flakes over each portion and place the cookie tray in freezer. Although two hours should be enough for it to freeze, but you may leave it for extra half an hour if you like it crunchier.
4) Serve as a frozen treat and enjoy the mouthwatering desert.

Nutritional Value per Serving

Calories 162

Carbohydrates 15 g

Protein 6 g

Total Fat 15 g

Icy Berry Banana Smoothie
Servings: 2

Cooking Time: 5 minutes

Ingredients

Frozen berries, 1 cup

Soymilk, 1 cup (vanilla flavored)

Bananas, 2 (medium sized)

Ice cubes

Method

1) In a food processor, whirl all ingredients for 3 minutes. Pulse more for a mother texture.
2) Add in ice cubes and pulse for another 30 seconds.
3) Whirl all the ingredients in a food processor, until smooth. You can also add a few ice cubes if you want.
4) Serve immediately or else the ice will melt and the smoothie will become watery!

Nutritional Value per Serving:

Calories 164.5

Carbohydrates 32 g

Protein 3.5 g

Total Fat 4.5 g

Cherry Brownies
Servings: 12

Cooking Time: 1 hour

Ingredients

Carob powder, ¼ cup

Dates, ½ cup

Dried cherries, ½ cup

Honey, 3 tablespoon

Walnuts, 1 cup

Method

1) In a blender, combine all ingredients and whirl until thoroughly blended.
2) Press the mixture into a (lightly greased) cake dish.
3) Place the dish in the freezer for about an hour or so. Do not over freeze it or else it will get difficult to slice it into smaller pieces.
4) Serve and enjoy the cherry brownies.

Nutritional Value per Serving

Calories 125

Carbohydrates 17.5g

Protein 2 g

Total Fat 6.4 g

Apricot with Cocoa Supreme
Servings: 12

Cooking Time: 5 minutes

Ingredients

Apricots, 2 cup (soaked in water for an hour)

Cocoa powder, 12 tablespoon

Ground flax seeds, ½ cup

Ground sunflower seeds, 1 cup

Sea salt, 2 teaspoon

Method

1) In a blender, pour in all ingredients, and pulse for 2 minutes or until everything is perfectly blended.
2) Serve immediately!

Nutritional Value per Serving

Calories 166

Carbohydrates 21.8 g

Protein 5.4 g

Total Fat 8.8 g

Berry Treat Smoothie
Servings: 4

Cooking Time: 5 minutes

Ingredients

Frozen strawberries, 1 cup

Frozen blueberries, 1 cup

Frozen raspberries, 1 cup

Frozen blackberries, 1 cup

Natural cherry juice, 2 cups

Vanilla bean yogurt, 2 cups (dairy free)

Method

1) In a food processor, pour in all the ingredients, and whirl until all berries are mixed and perfectly blended.
2) Once the smoothie is ready, pour the same amount of mixture into each serving glass and enjoy this healthy, yet yummy dessert.

Nutritional Value per Serving

Calories 120.5

Carbohydrates 26 g

Protein 2 g

Total Fat 1.2 g

Nutty Chocolate Gelato

Servings: 2

Cooking Time: 2 hours

Ingredients

Cocoa butter, 1 to 2 tablespoons

Coconut butter, 1 tablespoon

Coconut flakes, 2 tablespoons

Frozen bananas, 4

Liquid stevia, 10 drops (chocolate flavored)

Low fat coconut milk, ¼ cup

Pea protein powder, 1 scoop

Raw almond butter, 2 tablespoons

Method

1) Freeze peeled bananas in advance. Always freeze food items in a zip lock bag so that aroma of different flavors are not mixed with one another.
2) In a blender, combine frozen bananas along with cocoa powder, protein, coconut milk, almond butter, coconut butter, and stevia; and pulse until all ingredients are well mixed.
3) You may add a bit of more milk to make the mixture smoother. See your blender has an ice cream option. It is perfectly fine if there is no such option, just set it on highest level.
4) Pour the mixture into desert bowls and sprinkle some coconut flakes on each serving.
5) Place in the freezer for half an hour for delicious tasting gelato.

Nutritional Value per Serving

Calories 144

Carbohydrates 37 g

Protein 3 g

Total Fat 4 g